Walking Through Shattered Glass

With the help of my social media friends, I was able to break the barriers of Breast Cancer and come out on the Other Side.

Denice M. Duszynski

#1 Bestselling Co-Author of Empowered Women of

Social Media 1 and 2 and Chocolate & Diamonds for the

Woman's Soul "The Majesty of Motherhood"

Picking up the Pieces after Cancer

A Luna Claire Cute Little Book Publication
The Micro-Memoir ®
Published by Luna Claire Books
http://www.lunaclairebooks.com

Picking up the Pieces after Cancer

DEDICATION

To all who have got the diagnosis of Cancer and Survived, you are my hero. It's your fight that permits others to fight too. To my family who has been by my side through every treatment and every appointment. To my social media family, I couldn't have made it through without your love and light, prayers and uplifting of me during this journey.

Picking up the Pieces after Cancer

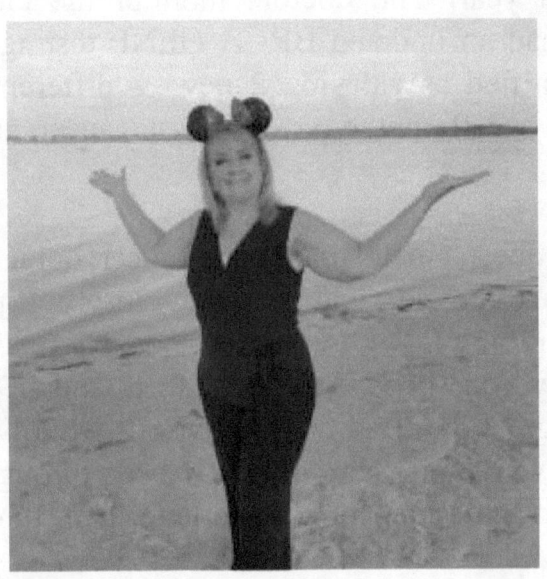

For 8 years now I've been cancer-free, and I plan on keeping it that way.

Treatments are necessary but not the way I want to live my life. My journey began the day after my treatments were done. For me, it's so important to put in my body everything to ward off anything that could trigger cancer. So, I began looking at my diet closely and learned everything I could about clean eating.

I became a label detective. I also know that our food is not the same as what our grandparents' food used to be. Our soil is depleted therefore our food is not nutritious.

Picking up the Pieces after Cancer

I continue to keep up my doctor's appointments and testing 3 times a year. The doctors monitor me closely. I've recently had an updated BRCA GENE testing. I've now been identified as carrying 2 new & different kinds of DNA for a different type of breast cancer and uterine cancer.

Now, this doesn't mean that I have cancer, but it does mean that I have to be alert and watching closely. It just means I'm carrying the DNA for those types. It's really good to know how your body functions, feels and if you're not having a great day find out the reasons why. For me, the biggest reward and everything I've been through is being able to advocate for women and help them through their journeys.

I found through the love of clean eating and holistic plants that I can teach people how to get the right nutrients into their bodies to help heal them. I teach cooking classes called Mermaid Dishes & also teach about how plants heal. It's really about learning how our bodies react to real food and to get rid of the Frankenstein foods. My motto is "Plants over Pills" to heal your body naturally.

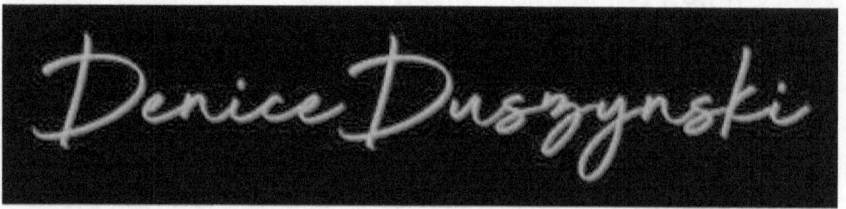

Walking through Shattered Glass

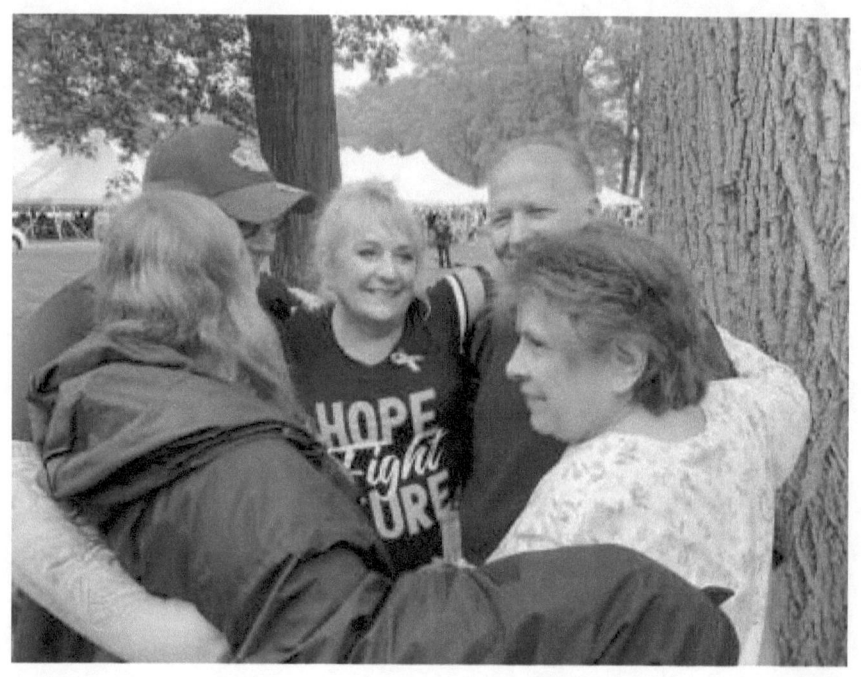

THE KEY TO HEALING IS IN FINDING SUPPORT FROM FRIENDS AND FAMILY.

MY STORY OF BEATING CANCER

Today I want to present this short book to you on how I made it through my diagnosis of cancer. It took me doing prayer and self-help work so very much but writing was one of the most cathartic experience that helped me truly find the truth of my power.

My first writing of this experience was published in a book called "Empowered Women of Social Media and this is my chapter. Today I am healthier and happier than I have ever been and want to encourage you that you can too. Take my advice and lean on your friends, let those who want to help you, help you, believe in your body's wisdom and how it is meant to heal itself. Mainly, trust GOD to get you through it. You can make it to the other side. I promise.

Today I thrive, and I want to help you thrive too. At the end of this book I will give you instructions on how to contact me and setup a time for us to have a good talk about what you are going through.

I can help you setup a program for your own body type that helps you continue making the necessary hormones and antibodies to keep your cells in optimal health. When you start to focus more on clean-food, and less on cancer, the cancer starts to flee from you.

Thank you for taking the time to read my book and I hope you will share it with others. It has been quite the unbelievable journey from then until now. I feel younger, more vibrant and healthier than I ever have at any other point in my life. I have 7 Grandchildren, am a great grandmother and have another grand baby on the way in October of 2019! WOO HOO.

Walking through Shattered Glass

Picking up the Pieces after Cancer

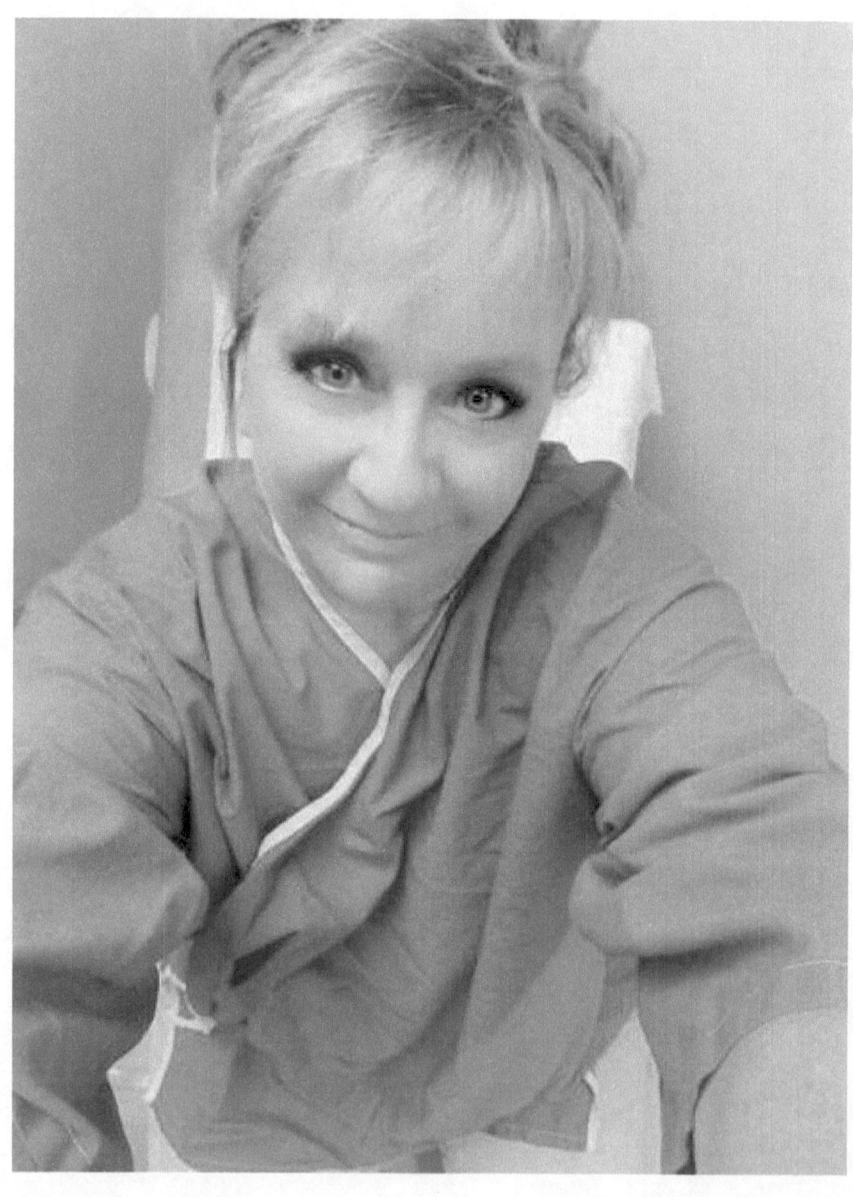

Walking through Shattered Glass

Picking up the Pieces after Cancer

PART ONE

DAILY STEPPING STONES

The Daily Facebook Saga

Daily Stepping Stones – The Facebook Saga

Life is a Daily Stepping Stone

My story is about learning to *live life living* no matter what comes your way. My journey begins the summer of 2011.

"Since the summer I had been having pains in my left arm and was visiting my chiropractor. He adjusted my back as I've had years of issues for several years from falling at an ice rink while skating. He said the area was in my heart area and he'd keep watch."

I continued with some minor medical issues during the summer thinking nothing of it. In late November on the plane ride from a conference in Las Vegas, by the way had the best time of my life meeting new people that fast became very close to me and I call very proud to call them my sisters and brothers, I began to experience bad pains.

My left arm became very sore and achy as well as my left breast. As soon as I got home, I started checking. "Oh my God! There's a lump!" I went a few days not saying anything to anyone because I kept thinking it's just a cyst (my body is prone to cysts). I got a wakeup call that day watching a medical show, saying call your doctor now.

I believe in my heart that it was divine intervention. It was now too late in the day to call and we are now into the Thanksgiving weekend. I finally told my husband and my mom. They were very concerned and encouraged me to move forward. So, first thing Monday morning I made the dreaded call.

I immediately went for a mammogram and an ultrasound. The radiologist said he found something and immediately sent me to a breast surgeon. My husband and I kept saying, "it will be ok" to each other, as we know my body throws cysts. Entering the surgeon's office, Dr. Keeney, it was surreal. She looked over my tests and knew right away.

Picking up the Pieces after Cancer

Having her sit there and saying to us "You have cancer," put me into shock. The words were numbing, knocking the wind from me. I thought I was prepared for whatever the doctor would say, but it's simple human nature to hope for the best. It really is that difficult to hear those words come out of your doctor's mouth.

My husband and I left the office in shock. We knew I had breast cancer, but our minds still could not wrap around what that really meant. Now I had to break it to my parents and children. As I did, they were in denial and had a lot of questions.

As it seeps into my mind, as I learn, research, talk to family and friends about it, they continue to be repeated thoughts.

Personal Note: These repeated thoughts are probably just like the ones you have had along your own journey.

"You need an operation…You need Chemo…You need radiation, too." And if you manage to get through it all, then you have little reminders creep up. "More blood work... You have a blood clot…We need to do another Mammo…Another Ultrasound. And, oh yeah, an MRI guided biopsy." It's seems at times to be never ending.

I needed to find a way to cope. I've always had a "just do it" and "it is what it is" attitude. I found my voice in journaling to myself in a private Facebook group when I found the lump. I start a new group in December called **Daily Stepping Stones**. This was the single best choice I made in finding a way to handle the cancer. It helped me keep an accurate record of what was going on daily in my life.

Using Facebook as a way to keep up with the journey is a great way to look back on your healing.

Picking up the Pieces after Cancer

Friends sent motivational sayings, offered prayers, and some interesting research, just in case I hadn't seen it! At the same time, I posted some of the research I found, sharing with my friends and family in the group. Every note or comment let me know I was not alone, and even better that I was very blessed with a loving, caring family and an amazing group of friends. Little did I know how well informed this would keep everyone and how much time, which was about to become a scarce commodity, it would save me. I was ready to do battle.

My journey over the next few years was probably much like any other cancer patient's journey, but the overwhelming love, positivity and hope that people extended to me, and still do, in real life, but especially on **Daily Stepping Stones**, really made a tremendous difference in how I looked at my days and weeks. I realized, by writing it out, that the details were just that, details. Ultimately though, I knew my family and friends and most important of all, that God had my back.

When I had enough strength, I would make my way to my computer on the other end of the house because I didn't have a tablet or a laptop at that time. If it was just 5 minutes, I wanted to connect with my friends and family daily. Every day I would find the time to post for my friends and to continue my business.

I LOVE YOU. CHECK YOUR BOOBIES!

One of the most important things I would do monthly, without fail, I reminded those I love to "Check your boobies." You can never check too often! It was exactly one year before that, I had a mammogram which showed nothing, so it's really important to do those monthly checks manually. During my battle, I learned of a 10-year-old girl who was diagnosed, and men get breast cancer, too.

My first procedure, a needle biopsy on my daughter's birthday, December 5th, was tolerable but scary and Dr.

Picking up the Pieces after Cancer

Keeney did a good job of numbing the area. I was sore and tried not to worry for the following week while waiting for the results. Next came an MRI, with dye contrast, which was told it could make me nauseous, but it didn't. While other's prepared for Christmas, I had meetings with doctors and specialists. It consumed my holiday spirit.

So now onto the information of the biopsy information. I'm very thankful for my support system as my Mom & daughter, Jessica went to the doctors with me. I needed them there to write all the information down about the cancer and necessary treatments as I'm having a hard time absorbing all the information.

The news – *Triple Negative Invasive Ductal Cancer* and the tumor is 1.5 cm. not currently showing anything in the lymph nodes. Dr. K told me when they did the surgery, they would put tracers into my sentinel nodes and remove at least two lymph nodes.

"I'm in stage 1 right now and will know more after they operate."

Our mutual hope is that I caught it early enough and I would stay at stage 1.

Between this day and my surgery date, December 29th, people on the Facebook page begin to reveal to me that they, too, were cancer survivors. I was so glad to hear their stories of survival. Prayers were literally pouring over me. I was offering up plenty of my own as well. The night before surgery was one of my tougher moments in this journey. I slept only three hours, never more than an hour at a time.

I was admitted at 9 A.M. and prepped for surgery. I had a blue space like suit to put on which was heated as was told patients do better when their bodies are warm. I was then injected with blue dye for the tracers at 10 o'clock, taken to the radiation active department to radioactive material injected into my breast and explained that my boob would turn blue and I might look a little blue gray for the day and pee like a smurf! A silent laugh and trying to keep my humor alive?

Next an IV was inserted with relaxation medication introduced. Dr. K arrived and explained to me of exactly what was going to happen step by step. A lumpectomy! I had the choice between a lumpectomy, but because I needed to return to work ASAP to keep my insurance going, I chose not to have the mastectomy.

I remember as they were getting ready to take me in for the operations turning to my Mom and husband, Paul and saying, "this isn't supposed to be happening to me" and whelming up with some fear of what was about to happen. I left the room with a smile, not letting my family know my fears.

I was now well relaxed from the meds and told the surgeon "let's get this over with." By 11:40, I was on the operating table, and I was told it would take approximately 90 minutes for the surgery. I wasn't keeping track of the time but trying to leaving in good spirits. My husband and mom asked the nurse if she could give me anesthesia as a daily supplement! More humor! I have cancer but not everyone has forgotten how to laugh.

Thank God for that because over the next year sometimes that was all we had. Surgery is simply the start.

By January 4, 2012, I posted that I was not feeling well, but my friends rallied with explanations: post-surgery funk? Sort of a detox of the anesthesia? In the next few days, I feel a little better, so tackle some chores and trying not to overdo it. It exhausts me and leaves me sore and swollen. Lesson learned.

My pathology results tell says they got all the cancer. I just need to check in with my doctor next week. Daily chores are difficult, but my energy appears to be returning. On the 8th I post another message:

I AM NOT MY BREAST CANCER

I am NOT my breast cancer.

27

Picking up the Pieces after Cancer

After reviewing my history, because I have breast cancer at the age of 50 and have triple negative cancer (disease that has not been fueled by estrogen, progesterone, and the HER-2/neu gene), there's a good chance that the insurance will cover all my testing. Apparently, there are 3 types of cancer. Sporadic (just by chance), Familial (caused by a combination of family & environment) and hereditary (occurs when an altered gene is passed down in the family). There's so much information to soak in. Mine is Sporadic.

My next appointment is a typical "good news, bad news" scenario. While unwrapping the bandages, I'm still swollen a lot. Although looking at my breast I'm thinking geeze, wasn't this supposed to be a lumpectomy? I'm realizing it's much more than just a lump removed it's more like a partial and I'm down at least 2 cup sizes.

I'm definitely lopsided! Ha ha ha ha!! They got all the cancer and the nodes showed NO cancer. The mass was a bit larger than the sonogram showed, so I actually had stage 2B cancer, the size of a walnut. I meet with technicians who will do "Oncotype" Testing to see exactly what type of cancer I have. I do some research realizing how important this is for choosing a course of treatment. Of course, that testing is two weeks off, and the waiting is always the worst.

My mother's cousin called in with information from her daughter which is a nurse "Sometimes flying will prompt conditions like this to come to the foreground because of the decompression and oxygen changes in flight."

I truly feel that a trip to Las Vegas saved my life. I had many obstacles to get there (mainly my workplace telling me I couldn't take 2 days off in a row because it is called extended holiday) (working in a school sometimes is hard) and if I had passed up that trip I may of been walking around for a while allowing my cancer to get worse.

Courage is not the towering oak that sees storms come and go; it is the fragile blossom that opens in the cold snow. Anonymous. So back to work full time just 2 weeks after my surgery and waiting on test results. I find the first half of my Oncotype testing indicates that I will not pass this cancer down through my family. This is really wonderful news!

Everyone around me is still holding me up, so I better hold myself up, too! Cancer is RUDE, OBNOXIOUS, & MEAN! But, so am I! So watch out cancer! **You have got one hell of a fight on your hands!**

The results of the pathology report. It is Triple Negative Invasive Ductal Cancer, an aggressive form which travels through the breasts milk ducts into the breast tissue and can infiltrate the lymph nodes and other parts of the body. It accounts for around 80% of the breast cancers diagnosed in women in the United States annually. It also carries a 10 to 20 percent risk of recurrence during a patient's lifetime. Not until you are cancer free for five years after treatment, can you truly know that you are cancer free.

On January 24th Dr. K tells me I need to have a port put in, but there is some delay. Meanwhile next Tuesday, I have to go for lab work; then a MUGA Scan, which will determine part of my heart's ability to undergo toxic chemotherapy; then a premeeting with Pam, Dr. Scalzo's nurse for a "Teach Class", so I will know everything that will happen. It is what it is, and I will do what I have to do, even though it will not be pleasant. I type Peace & Love to you all. Though typed through tears, I feel like have no choice.

February arrives quickly, with Chemo knocking on my door. Got the call to have the port put in. Dr. Scalzo expedites that as he is anxious for me to get started with Chemo. On February 8th, with a Valium and local anesthetic, in 40 short minutes, my port is in, thanks to the Nurse Practitioner at Dr. Scalzo's office. Messages of hope fill my Daily Stepping Stones page: for a smooth procedure; a good night's sleep; prayers, always prayers; some ironically posted at the exact time I am having a procedure.

Picking up the Pieces after Cancer

It's comforting to know that someone was thinking of me at a moment when I was scared or in pain. Loving messages of consolation follow with inquiries as to how I am feeling? I'm very thankful for Social Media. Connecting with people I otherwise would have never met. I've now met many of these wonderful people in person.

Finally, I meet Dr. Scalzo, who is very kind and caring. He speaks to me on my level and answers all my questions. His news: I will have at least 5 months of Chemo, first 4 infusions consist of Adriamycin and Cytoxan, the red Kool-Aid looking stuff that makes your hair fall out, infusions are every other week, followed by an injection of Neulasta to boost my white blood count. I am told I will have my chemo infusions on Fridays, then shots on Saturdays. My daughter is an LPN and has volunteered to give them to me.

Anti-nausea scripts today, since I will likely be nauseated for 2-3 days after the sessions and feel fatigued. I soon find out that is an understatement. By the 2nd infusion, I'm so sick and can barely get out of bed. If you've ever had the flu, it's 20 times worse and the constipation is so bad. Eating is a priority, but food literally makes me sick. I can't seem to get fluids down me either.

When the first 8 weeks are up, I will be put on another chemo drug called Taxol for 12 weeks. These are weekly treatments and I'm told this will be a much easier infusion. The chemo treatment should end towards the end of end of June. Then I will have 5 weeks of daily radiation, plus one week of what they refer to as a boost. After the first week of chemo, my hair will probably start to fall out. So I will be looking for a shorter hairstyle in the next week. My determination is still unshakable. I refuse to post anything negative and only keep thinking positive thoughts.

My daily affirmations and posts are important. *I will remember that to find the joy in rainbows, I must endure the rain.* And I will remember always that while I may have Cancer, Cancer does not have me! And then, having a positive attitude is the best medicine for cancer! I will never let it get me down. I will stand up and fight this horrible monster!" All the encouragement, with stories and experiences of others continue to come in on Facebook group. People ask for my snail mail address. I am feeling loved.

SMILE - it will make you look better! PRAY - it will keep you Stronger! LOVE - it will make you Enjoy Life!

A few days later, my daily affirmation empowers me again. God only puts things in our life that he thinks we're strong enough to handle. He has given me many trials throughout my life, and this is the biggest battle ever! God must think I'm pretty strong. I will kick Cancers butt! I post positively, but realistically this time. Being happy doesn't mean that everything is perfect. It means that you've decided to look beyond the imperfections. Author Unknown.

I asked that my friends on Daily Stepping Stones start a prayer chain as my chemo is getting ready to start. My Chemo starts today, *February 17th*, and will take three – four hours for each infusion. I feel the prayer chain working. Thank God for Facebook, it keeps me connected to everyone posting on my progress and certainly can't thank them individually or even enough for their prayers and positive reinforcements. I certainly never could have guessed the tremendous amount of help I would receive from this close circle of about seventy friends, plus over 10,000 people through Social Media who are following my daily progress. As my husband and my mom drives me to my first appointment it's a blur, but I do remember asking God to get me through this in prayer.

My energy plummets and the nausea start. Everyone constantly remind me that God and Angels are surrounding and protecting me. These are just the early days, but I am thankful for so much, this week, I'm particularly thankful for my anti-nausea medication.

Picking up the Pieces after Cancer

Dr. Keeney wants to keep me out of work longer and I agree. I'm so ill that I can barely make the walk into her office. Labs and checkups the following day go well with Dr. Scalzo. My blood cell counts are down. I talk to Dr. Scalzo my oncologist about this and right from the beginning he didn't want me going back to work. Working at a school with children and adults during sick season would definitely make my health worse. I'm taking no chances and I'm out of work for the remainder of my treatment.

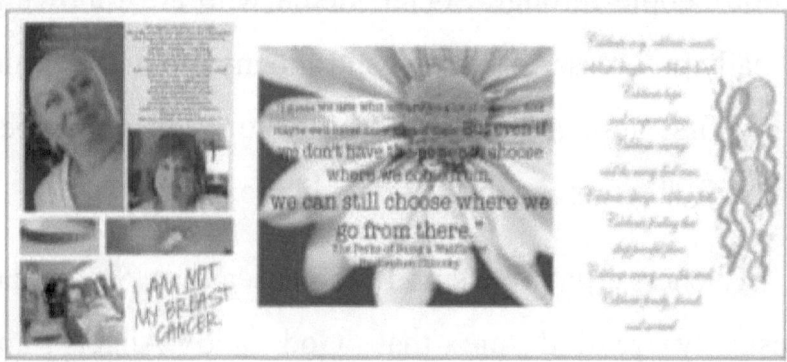

The uplifting messages on **Daily Stepping Stones** continue, I thank God every day for Social Media. I get to meet people from all over the world that I would never have got to meet. I went to the American Cancer Society and attended their 'Look Good, Feel Good' program. They taught us the techniques of how to apply make-up after hair loss, tie scarves not just for your head, but for your body, too. I also learn cancer hygiene, things on how to cleanse my breath and control medical/medicinal body odor. Thanks ACS. You rock!

It didn't take long for the chemo to start killing every cell in my body. On March 1st I got up to take care of my hair. Did you just hear me SCREAM? My hair is starting to fall out!!!!! Just when needed an uplifting moment, I get a special surprise from Carol Baldwin from the Baldwin Cancer Foundation. She's also is the mom to those famous son's, the Baldwin Brothers. Yep, you know who they are, right! It's a big Pink Hug, a beautiful pink plush blanket with a handwritten note from Carol. Wow, that is so special, and tears of joys were expressed. Beth Baldwin, daughter of Carol, also asked for my number and calls me later that day. She knows my struggles that I may not be able to pay my insurances. Beth tells me "She is looking into options for my insurance but… not to worry about it and let it go and put it into God's hands. I will not have to pay those extreme costs it's going to cost me.

$1500 a month for my insurance." What an amazing and caring couple of women! It's just hard with no disability insurance and wondering how on earth we are going to pay for everything.

That very same week, my daughter surprises me that she's been working on a benefit to help me pay for my insurance. Strike Out Cancer – A bowling benefit. Circulars announcing a benefit bowl-a-thon to help me through this time, go out. It's scheduled for April 1st. My husband's company also joins in on the benefit and puts on a benefit luncheon for their employees. Whatever the employees pay for their lunch, the company matches. Some even threw in their whole weekly paycheck. I'm so thankful and grateful for this, as all of my insurance is now covered and some of my outstanding medical bills will be covered too.

Walking through Shattered Glass

I just got a call from my Dr. Scalzo's office. My lab results showed that my calcium has skyrocketed, which can be dangerous. It is March 6th, and in hindsight, the calcium news was sort of forgotten at the moment. I now had to make a decision which is one of the hardest things I've ever done in my life. My hair was coming out in globs in my brush and I was literally suffocating from the hair falling around me.

My daughter brought the clippers over and now I'm bald! Yes, it will start growing out again in 4 -5 months, but you really don't know how it feels until you must do something so far out of your realm of possibilities. It was truly on a par with the emotional kick in the chest the original delivery of my cancer diagnosis held. And just when I thought it couldn't get worse, I couldn't sleep. The stubble on my head hurt just like every inch of my body is so tender from the chemo. It destroys every cell in your body. So, two days later my daughter came to shave it clean. I'm a cue ball.

Picking up the Pieces after Cancer

I try to stay positive at every turn, I truly do. But shaving my head seemed like the worst thing, so maybe it was a good turning point when I look back. No one shunned me or acted embarrassed to be with me. Revelation: If I am not my cancer, I am certainly not my hair!

Time passes, with "little setbacks". The sky-high calcium was actually bottomed out Vitamin D (Vitamin D is a hormone that is linked to breast cancer, so I find out. Please everyone gets your Vitamin D check right away.), and skin irritations, fatigue, nausea. Cancer is a full-time job. But at the end of my day, I always have one place to seek solace: my *Daily Stepping Stones*. A new chemo, a fake boob (the girl fitting me asked my husband to feel it, much to his embarrassment), and the news that I can't exercise arrive because my heart rate goes up over 200 just from walking into his office. Honestly, did a doctor actually see me dragging my butt in here and think I was fatigued from too much exercise? New glasses are picked out, pink and purple, of course.

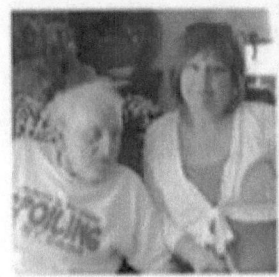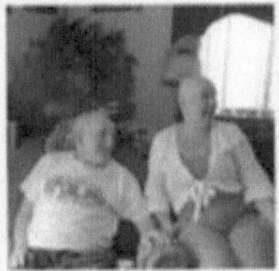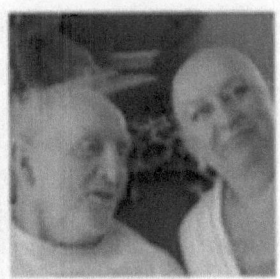

I just had to share this picture. I stopped at my Dad's to give him his Father's Day card and to get pictures. I rarely go anywhere at this point of the game and this is the first time I've ventured out to anywhere other than the doctors and chemo sessions. I feel so isolated from the world, so I'm blessed that social network allows me to be able to connect with people. Can't get their germs that way. So, in the middle of pictures, I pulled off my wig. I told my mom I needed a picture of the two baldies but seems my Dad does have more hair than me now. Lol I don't let anyone see me like this, but the dogs were on my mom's lap and just stared at me like what the hell did you just do. It was funny and we laughed. Even my Dad laughed! Oh yeah and I had a red wig on, and I don't do red. That was my husband's Father's Day gift. He was begging me to wear it for months. Now I can put that one away!

June rolls around and I start thinking about my days when the Chemo will be finally finished. I can't wait to get out of bed and do all the things that most people take for granted and my bucket list is building. A cruise, shopping, NYC, travel and so much more. Through all of this journey, I focused on my business and social networking instead of my illness. I truly know that because I had something as simple as Facebook and Social Media to go to daily, it saved my life.

On one hand, all I want is for my chemo…my cancer…this entire experience to be over, but some things in life become even more important than dealing with Cancer. I postponed one of my last Chemo treatments to attend my youngest son, Cody's high school graduation. The last of my babies to graduate from high school. What a beautiful sight to see him with his maroon colored cap and gown. I'm crying and celebrating with the class of

2012. This year had been extremely rough on him and I'm so relieved that we both have made it this far.

Hello July 2nd, and yes, thank you! My last Chemo! As I get set up for my final round of infusions, I get the typical health questions. I answered yes to a swelling in my ankle. And of course, never a dull moment, a blood clot is detected in my left leg after a Doppler is performed. So, before I leave, I get a shot of Lovenox and a script for Coumadin. I now have to give myself daily shots. Again, Social Media saves the day. I search out how to give myself a shot because I don't want to be a burden to my family anymore.

It's time to finish up and get the last chemo done. I always say a prayer before my chemo's and ask God to keep me safe. I have seen so many taken out by ambulance due to a chemo reaction. It's finally over!!

I am relieved that I made it through and though the following weeks are tough, I am feeling better and better, little by little every day! It took 4 weeks to get my taste buds back. My follow up July 19th, with the Dr. Scalzo with a lot of fantastic news. I don't have to see a vascular surgeon; my port is being removed on July 31st and they APPROVED me to start taking a Fiber supplement to help me lose weight. Dr. Scalzo said it is a good thing for me to be taking right now since the chemo is over. He was impressed with my all-natural approach for healing the body and losing weight. I really need the digestive enzymes to get my stomach issue taken care of and flush those toxins out.

It's July 27th and I have made it through my first week of radiation and it has gone well, though I am warned it can get tough when I start to "Sun-Burn. Oh, and I might be fatigued! (Feel free to insert your own laugh here.)

Never a month passes without a reminder to "Do your boobie check!" People simply must check their breasts. It can be the matter between life and death. I love all the support but if I have helped one person get through their journey with this message alone is the only purpose of my Daily Stepping Stones and on Social Medias, I will have accomplished my goal.

August 17th, Just an update on my progress. Today is #18 of 30 radiations. So far, I'm doing well…Here's to each of you for standing by me, encouraging me, and being my friend during the journey. I will have many stories to come I'm sure.

September 2012 Thanks so much for all of your support, cyber hugs, and prayers. I will keep you updated. As I close out the evening and prepare for tomorrow, (back to school) I just wanted to tell you how awesome it is to have this group. During my illness this past year, it has inspired me to keep forging ahead and motivates me knowing that I can help you. I want to thank everyone from the bottom of my heart for getting me through my daily struggles.

The summer has flown, and tomorrow is September 3, I return to work. It's a big day for me. I haven't completed my treatment and I'm returning to work today so my insurance will kick in. Today is the last day of radiation. Here I am lying in the radiation room about to receive the final treatment. The radiation machine is so big and scary. I'm so glad it's over. I did have a minor rash from the radiation and that is where I seem to be peeling. I'm feeling good, just a little fatigued. This week I have two physicals coming up... one with my Gyno and one with my general doctor.

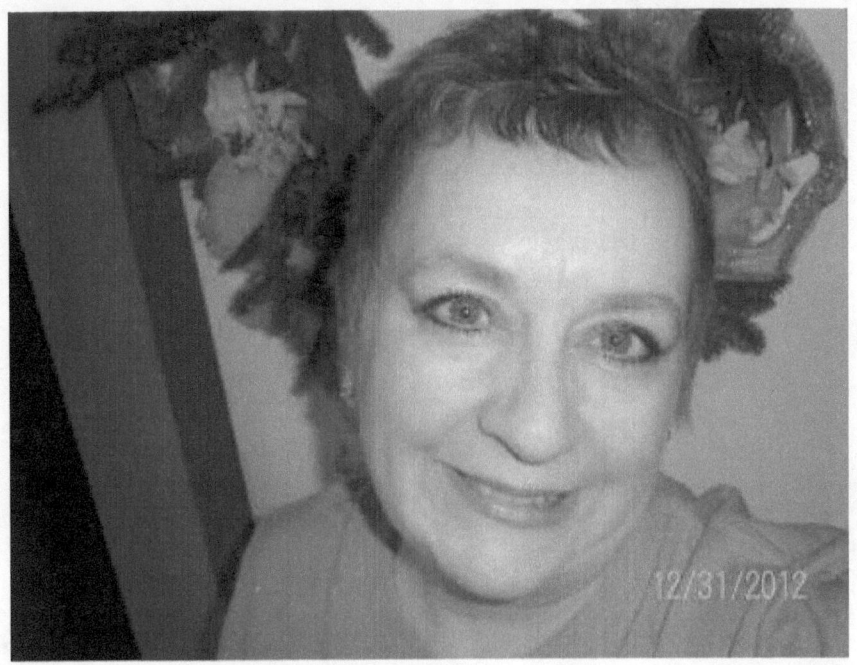

This is a photo of me when my hair was just starting to grow back in 2012. I think that keeping a smile on my face was one of the best ways I was able to make it through.

Picking up the Pieces after Cancer

October 25th, I go to see the Radiologist for a checkup. My only real complaint is incessant fatigue, but it is just a side effect from the radiation. I've posted a few times in between but less about cancer and more about life, and business. I think this is a good sign!

In early November, I head to the Lymphedema Clinic for physical therapy. Chemo and radiation effects are starting to take a toll on my body. Possibly its arthritis setting into my joints in my legs, hips, and hands. Some days I can hardly walk as it's getting so painful. Also, the tissue in my arm pit and around to my back is starting to stiffen up even with the stretching exercises. I had a deep scapula massage yesterday which seemed to help.

November 18, 2012, I had my two month check last week with Dr. Scalzo. My labs came back and all my levels are normal. My breast check was normal too! I pray every day that my healing will continue, and cancer will NEVER return.

Within the next month or so, I find out that one of my supporters through this journey, has been diagnosed and another is being checked for a suspicious spot. They are going through the same struggles of breast cancer and need our support to **Daily Stepping Stones** to give them the support they will need in the coming months. I invite my beautiful friends and supporters. I can tell you this is certainly a post I hoped I would never have to make. It would have been enough for me to have gone through it.

December 12th has arrived and I'm heading for my 3-month check with my breast surgeon today. I can't believe that a year ago I found out I had breast cancer. What a year it's been! She says that all looks well, no lumps or bumps. I ask if I can have the Thermography mammogram for my check-up, instead of a traditional Mammo? I don't want any more radiation in my body! Radiation is a carcinogen itself. Dr. Keeney agrees. Unfortunately, there is no one local and insurance doesn't cover it so traditional approach is the only way now. It is important to take an active role in your health care. I will also have to have a breast MRI in June.

December 27th, 2013 Just got a call from Cancer Connects Wellness Clinic and I got my massages approved...having issues with my left arm...which is probably from Lymph nodes being removed a year ago...same pain that I had just before I found out I had cancer...hoping it's just the lymph nodes over reacting from all the holiday cheer we've had over the last few weeks.

January 5, 2013. Is it really 2013? Talk about a reality check? I just saw this article and it made me realize there is something much worse than my cancer and that of my adult friends. The article, titled: "Post Traumatic Stress for Parents of Children with Cancer" is so informative and a must for parents.

http://www.cancer.org/cancer/news/news/parents-of-kids-with-cancer-suffer-posttraumatic-stress

January 18th, Praise Jesus! My mammogram went well today, and no cancer was found! I'm now 4 months FREE!

March 19th today is my 6-month checkup. Labs early this morning and seeing Dr. Scalzo at 4pm. It's definitely a journey. I knew when I started, it was so surreal, and I thought it was never going to end. Here I sit today; my hair is about 1 inch long; my breasts are lopsided. Lol, and I now wear a prosthesis; and I have neuropathy in my feet and hands. But God I'm alive now, on the inside and out!

April 26th, 2013 just had my 7-month checkup. Doc says everything is looking good!! Those that have been following, thanks for the prayers and keeping me motivated through the last year. Having breast cancer last year certainly wasn't easy and it wasn't in my plans. It is a journey and I have met so many wonderful people. May God bless you all!

July 27th, 2013 had my 10-month check on Wednesday/Thursday! I'm still struggling with blood clots in my left leg and have a severe pain in my right arm. But I feel pretty good and on my way to a cancer free life!

August 21st, 2013 Went for my breast MRI this morning. Pray that I'm free of Cancer. It's been almost a year since my last chemo/radiation treatments.

August 22nd, 2013, well setbacks do occur, but at least the setbacks are not cancer and I beat cancer. My body continues to break down and I truly believe it's from the chemo treatments. So, I report arm pain, thinking its tendonitis, but it maybe tears in my rotator cuff that will take me out of work for 4 months. Again, no disability benefits, but I'm thankful for my home-based business. I will not let this get me down!!!

I am a fighter! Surgery scheduled for November 1st. The surgeon is supposed to stretch the muscle and fold it over and put a screw into the muscle and bone. I had a wonderful healing from God the day before. When the surgeons got into the shoulder, they could only find some fraying and scraped some arthritis. Just a few weeks of physical therapy and I'm back to normal

February 27, 2014. What a jump in time! That is definitely good news, but on the not so good side I am going thru a little crap right now. Found a lump a few weeks ago. I had a stat mammogram, then an ultrasound. Radiologist says it's a pocket of fluid and sends me for an MRI with contrast. I saw my breast surgeon yesterday; she felt the abnormality so did an ultrasound. She wants to send me to get an MRI guided biopsy. I can tell you I was pretty upset when I left her office. I don't want to go thru all this again.

February 28th, My MRI guided biopsy is scheduled for next Tuesday. The technicians tried 5 times to get the IV in my arm and hand, but it keeps rolling out. I'm well hydrated and they had 3 people try to get it inserted. To me it's confirmation from God that I don't need it. They provided another ultrasound and it doesn't show it growing in comparison from the MRI I had last week. My team of doctors are taking good care of me and watching closely.

On April 3rd, I had a follow up with my Breast Surgeon, Dr. Keeney yesterday. She reminded me that we still need to keep a close watch and made me promise to have an ultrasound in six months.

Three years later, it's now August 12 and I have another blood clot, flying home from Las Vegas convention that I just got through speaking at. I just got to tell everyone about my breast cancer journey, how a daily routine and Social Media saved my life. Everything is coming full circle for me. I am focusing on my home-based business and continuing my leave with the school district. Little problems pop up and I know all I have to do is go to my social network for love and support. Today I am alive, cancer free and happy. I am thriving, my business is thriving, and my family and friends are still exactly where I want them...in my life. My motto! Live Life Living!

Could I have done without it all? Yes! But I still believe that everything happens for a reason. I believe in the greatness of God and his ability to judge just how much you can handle. He's always there for you and loves you through the toughest of times.

Some days I may question it all, but then think God had a plan and is planning my next journey. I have love and I did handle it with Grace and the Empowerment of God. I will never forget that I am one of the ones who are truly blessed.

Girls can CHANGE the WORLD

CANCER WILL NEVER WIN BECAUSE WE WILL NOT LET IT WIN!

PART TWO THE LOOKING GLASS CHAPTER OF LIFE AFTER CANCER

THE LOOKING CLASS OF CANCER: THE LIES, BETRAYAL AND THE HEALING

Many survivors of cancer consider their lives to be a blessing. I am not implying that others do not see their lives in this way, but when you have stared death in the face and survived; every day that you are given feels extra special. I have undergone so many emotional, physical, and spiritual transformations since my journey has begun. I have often said that I feel like "Alice in Wonderland," looking at my life through a looking glass. It has truly been a surreal experience.

I've always been the kind of person who embraces life experiences, but I did not know how to cope when I heard the words, "You have cancer." My life was turned upside down instantly.

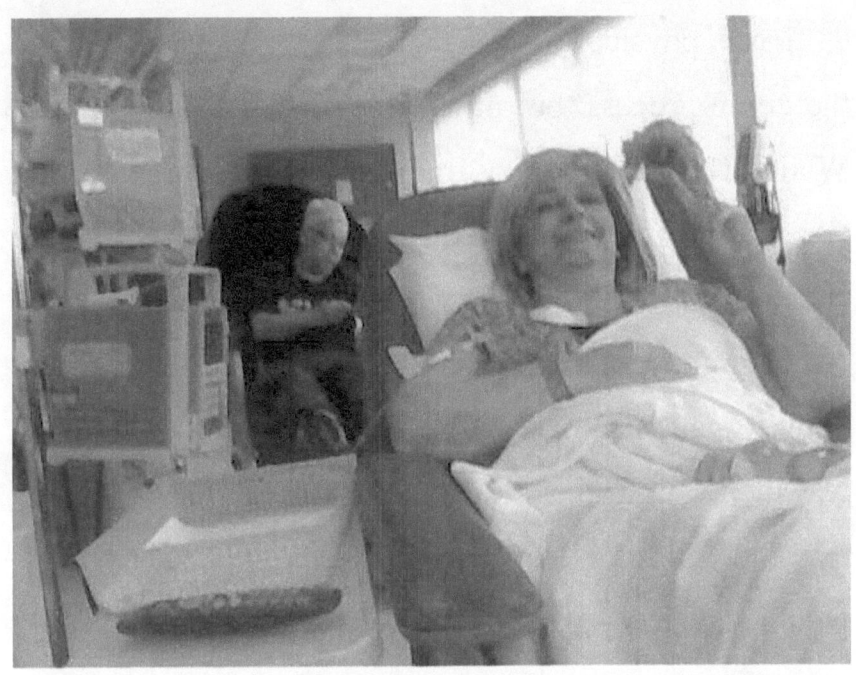

During the process, I was bombarded with invasive tests, to find out exactly what type of cancer it was. Within the first 30 days of finding the lump in my breast, I had blood tests, a needle biopsy, mammograms, ultrasounds and MRIs with dye contrasts. Oh, and did I say more blood tests? My body was invaded with needles, radioactive materials, surgical knives, and IVs. I endured this just so that they could remove one stupid walnut sized tumor.

Picking up the Pieces after Cancer

I was physically and emotionally exhausted through the entire process, but my journey had only just begun. While I was healing from the first surgery (the lumpectomy), they inserted a port into my chest for the chemotherapy. I did chemo weekly for five months. I spent grueling hours of having magic toxins going through my body to get every last invading cancer cell. Although it was something that was greatly needed, it left me extremely ill for at least five days each week. Just when I would start feeling better on day six and seven, I would start all over again with another round of chemo.

During this time, I lost my sense of taste and smell. I also felt like I was losing my mind. It destroyed my bone marrow for the first four sessions, and I needed shots weekly to rebuild it. Sometimes it's hard to grasp the fact that all of that has happened to me. I was the healthy one in my family. I taught good nutrition, exercise, and a healthy lifestyle. I never smoked, and I rarely had a glass of wine or any other alcohol. I would often think, how could this be my life?

During that horrible time in my life I had some support from my family, and I am eternally grateful for the love and care that they showed me. However, it seemed like most of my friends forgot me. The people that I have been there for were nowhere to be found in my time of need. My saving grace was social media. I gathered a lot of my strength through social media worldwide. What is funny is that I started using social media in 2006 to for Farmville because my friends were playing it. It was fun but very time-consuming and addicting. I took my crops seriously, and I would like to believe that I had one awesome farm. What started out as a simple hobby became so much more.

I started to meet people on Facebook that I would never have had the opportunity to meet otherwise. Social media has a way of connecting us all and because of the connections that I built; I had a support system to get me through the worst of my days.

I have a tight-knit and a large circle of friends who would check on me and help me get through the day. I thank God for them. My friends from all over the world would stop by, giving me encouragement and comfort through their words. It is amazing how many people you have never met face to face care about you. Many would private message me and ask questions as they were about to embark on their very own journey. I would calm them with thoughts of hope and faith and even pray with them. I am so honored to be able to comfort others while I was going through my own trials.

Following the cancer treatment, I began radiation. My chemotherapy was over, and it was time for me to go back to work so that my health insurance could be reinstated. I had to go back to my job because cancer is not cheap. It was extremely overwhelming to be working with children with disabilities. The long grueling hours took a toll on me physically, emotionally and mentally. I knew I could not do the job anymore.

During that time, I explored other options and continued to focus on me and my new career, my online business, and used every spare moment building a new career I was able to establish a new career through social media and it was a Godsend, a divine intervention. It prepared me for the biggest breakthrough I've ever had. I had a ton of support and love from mostly women around the world on social media and within six months my business started to flourish.

What I had worked so hard for finally came to fruition. My business exploded. Every break, every lunch, getting up two hours before I had to go to that job, heading to the bathroom with phone in hand just to take 5 minutes to answer a question or check in on social media, it was worth it all. I would come home and spend my time on social media until I was exhausted and needed to sleep.

Building relationships with people from Facebook and other media was vital to my success. I vowed never to go back to that job.

Picking up the Pieces after Cancer

Late winter, 2014, I found another lump in my breast. A bit panicky I called my oncologist. I went in immediately for examination. He confirmed there was something there. I headed right over for a stat mammogram and ultrasounds. Yikes, yes there was something there, but further test were needed. After visiting my breast care surgeon, she ordered a stat MRI Guided Needle Biopsy with contrast die so they could get a better look at the mass and take a sample.

The morning I went for the MRI I was a wreck. All the feelings of what I went through with cancer were flooding back. I really didn't want to go through this process all over again. Multiple people within the clinic tried to start my IV, but it continued to roll out. It was extremely painful and frustrating; no one could get it right. Eventually I said, "no way, you are done." The nurse asked my permission to bring in the other nurse. I said I didn't want it, but reluctantly agreed to at least have them look. The nurse came in, and I have had him before. I knew he was good and but still I was very nervous. He promised me he would not do the procedure unless he was confident, he could get the vein.

So, I agreed. Again, with no luck and the needle rolled out. I let him attempt a second time, with no luck. So, they asked if the head guy could come in and just look. By that time, I was crying heavily because it was so stressful and painful. So, he came in, took a look and said the only other way was to send me to the hospital and have a surgical procedure to have a PICC line put in. I flat out refused.

I told them this was God's way of telling me I did not need this. I was not having that procedure. So, they again asked permission to discuss with the unit doctor, to have an ultrasound done to take a look. I was ok with that as it was not so invasive. While sitting with the head nurse in her office trying to compose myself with my husband, we found she was a child of God. She chatted with us about her story.

I somehow think this day was a divine intervention. She excused herself from her office to see if my room was ready. My husband and I sat there and heard a noise behind us. The noise was like a metal door opening. We turned around, and there was a locker door ajar. On this locker door was a sign. "my life is BLESSED" My husband and I just looked at each other. We knew it was a sign from God everything would be okay.

When the nurse returned, we told her what had happened. She said that was her locker, and it is always shut. We knew it was a God experience. My name is Denice Duszynski and this is my story, there is life before cancer and there is life after cancer.

Social media is an important part of my life today. I started using social media in 2006 for Farmville because my friends were playing it, it was fun but very time consuming. Since then I have undergone many life transformations. Emotional, physical and spiritual transformations, yes many changes.

I feel like *"Alice in Wonderland"*, looking at my life through a looking glass. It really is a surreal experience. I know I'm supposed to embrace life experiences, but I keep thinking of how things really were, hearing those words, "You have cancer!" then your whole life in an instant is turned upside down.

You're bombarded with tests, and I mean invasive tests, to find exactly what type of cancer it is. Within the first 30 days of finding the lump in my breast, I had blood tests, needle biopsy, mammograms, ultrasounds, MRI's with dye contrast and did I say more blood tests. Your body is invaded with needles, radioactive material, surgical knives, IV's all just to remove the lump... that stupid walnut sized tumor.

Then the real fun begins. While I was healing from the first surgery, the lumpectomy, which was more like a partial as my breast is half the size it was, they inserted a port for the chemo. Mind you, they did all this to save my life. Once the port was inserted into my chest the chemo began, weekly for 5 months. I spent grueling hours of having this magic toxin going into my body, to get every last invading cancer cell.

This process left me vomiting, constipated, weak and very ill for at least 5 days each week. I would just start feeling a little better on day 6 and 7 just to start the process all over again with another round of chemo. My thoughts left me as well as smell and taste. It destroyed my bone marrow for the first 4 sessions, and I needed shots weekly to rebuild it. I'm still looking back at this travesty while trying to move forward. This was never supposed to happen to me. I was the healthy one in the family, teaching good nutrition, exercise and living a healthy lifestyle. I never smoked and rarely have a glass of wine or other alcohol. I thank God for my friends from all over the world would stop by, giving me encouragement and comfort through their words. It's amazing how many people you've never met face to face really care about you.

Many would private message me and ask questions as they were about to embark on their very own journey. I would calm them with thoughts of hope and faith and even pray with them. I'm so honored to be able to do that.

Oh, did I tell mention how horrible the side effects were? Every stitch of hair on my body was gone in the first 3 weeks of chemo. I was bald as a cue ball and it hurt both physical and emotionally.

You wouldn't believe how losing my hair like this literally made my scalp scream in pain. I wore soft caps to keep my head warm and protect as it was very sensitive. My eyebrows, lashes, pit and pubic hair was all gone. No leg hair. I was smooth as a baby.

My walking heart rate rose to over 200 which is very dangerous, so I started using a wheelchair. Then the blood clots started in my leg. Liver function started to decline. A constant watch for lymphedema still plagues me. My hands and feet still have remnants of neuropathy in them. 5 months into the treatment I had a week's break and then I received a 37 daily regiments of radiation –I was given measurements on where to exactly lay, tattooed for perfect alignment, burning and extreme tiredness. All this for what- oh yes, to save my life.

So, with all the cancer treatment behind me, I started moving forward – looking into the other side of the looking glass. Trying to see a new life and new future.

During this time, I had some support from my family. Seems like most of my friends locally forgot me. I gathered a lot of my strength through social media worldwide. I have a tight knit and large circle of social media friends who would check on me daily and help me get through the day.

I thank God for them. My friends from all over the world would stop by, giving me encouragement and comfort through their words.

During my radiation treatments, I went back to my full-time job at school to reinstate my health insurance. It's was a rough 9 months, but things were going well. During the cancer treatment I had to go on family leave from my J.O.B, you know what that stands for right? Just over

Broke!!! Well my JOB made me even broker. As a Teaching Assistant working for the state, during family leave there is NO disability insurance.

So, it was imperative I find a way to bring in income because CANCER is NOT CHEAP.

Following the cancer treatment, it was extremely overwhelming to be working with children with disabilities. The long grueling hours took a toll on me physically, emotionally and mentally. I knew I couldn't do this job anymore. It's hard when you have no support at work. Every day I left with tears running down my face. I was allowed to be abused, beaten up, and the students could do or say anything until someone gets hurt.

The school system was broke and it broke me. I continued to focus on me and my new career, my online business, using every spare moment. Building a new career through social media was a God send, a divine intervention. It prepared me for the biggest break through I've ever had. I had so much support and love from mostly women around the world on social media and within 6 months my business started to flourish. What I had worked for so hard, finally came to fruition. My business exploded. It was worth my time.... every break, every lunch, getting up two hours before I had to go to that job, heading to the bathroom with phone in hand just to take five minutes to answer a question or check in on social media.

I would come home and spend my time on social media until I was exhausted and needed to sleep. Building relationships with people of Facebook and other Medias was so important to my success.

I vowed never to go back to that job. Unfortunately, as my business was taking off, I had minor shoulder surgery just as school was starting. Yet again the chemo had broken down my body a little more.

Late winter, 2014, I found another lump in my breast. A bit panicky I called my oncologist. I went in immediately for examination. He confirmed there was something there. I headed right over for a stat mammogram and ultrasounds. Yikes... yes there is something there, but further test were needed. After visiting my breast care surgeon, she ordered a stat MRI Guided Needle Biopsy with contrast die so they could get a better look at the mass and take a sample.

The morning I went for the MRI I was a wreck. All the feelings of what I went through with cancer were flooding back. I really didn't want to go through this process all over again.

So, the nurse came out to get me started for the procedure, they had to start an IV, so reluctantly I went into the cold and sterile room. The first nurse tried to start the IV and it rolled out. I told her she only got one chance with a little scared laughter and nervously shaking with tears welling up. She promised me if she didn't think she could get it this time, she would get a nurse that was an expert in it. So, she proceeded and said she was confident she found a vein that would work. Well guess what!! No, it didn't work and the IV rolled right out again. I'm like "no way, you're done." She asked my permission to bring in the other nurse. I said I didn't want it, but reluctantly agreed to at least have them look.

The nurse came in and I've had him before. I knew he was good and but still I was very nervous. He promised me he wouldn't do the procedure unless he was confident, he could get the vein.

So, I agreed. Again, with no luck and the needle rolled out. I let him attempt a second time, with no luck. So, they asked if the head guy could come in and just look. By now I was crying heavily because it was so stressful and painful. So, he came in took a look and said the only other way was to send me to the hospital and have a surgical procedure to have a surgical iv **picc** put in. I flat out refused. I told them this was Gods way of telling me I didn't need this. I wasn't having this procedure.

They once again asked permission to discuss with the unit doctor, to have an ultrasound down to take a look. I was ok with that as it's not so invasive. While sitting with the head nurse in her office trying to compose myself with my husband, we found she was a child of God. She chatted with us about her story. I somehow think this day was a divine intervention.

She excused herself from her office to see if my room was ready. My husband and I sat there and heard a noise behind us. The noise was like a metal door opening. We turned around and there was a locker door ajar. On this locker door was a sign. "my life is BLESSED" My husband and I just looked at each other.

We knew it was a sign from God everything would be OK. When the nurse returned, we told her what had happened. She said that was her locker and it is always shut. We knew it was a God experience.

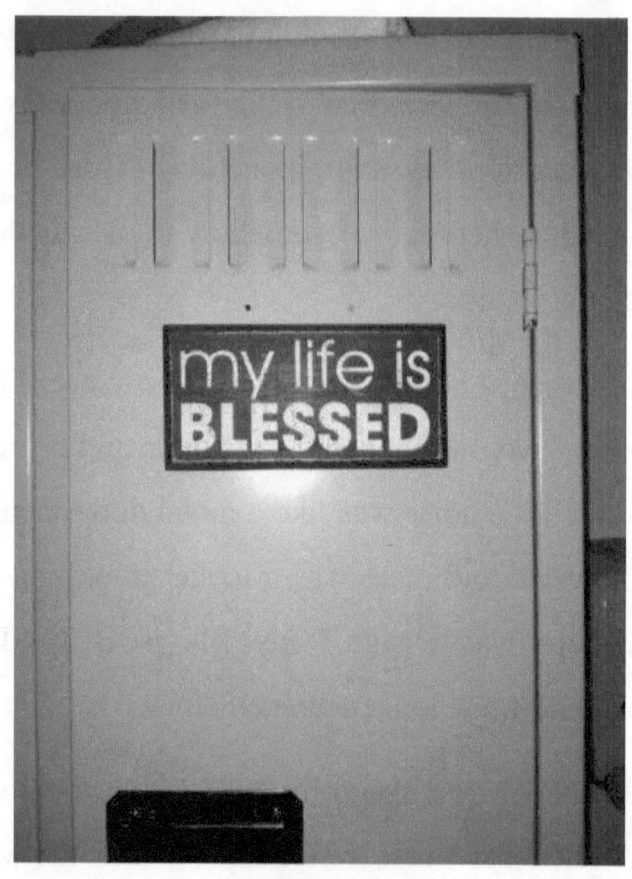

My business grew at an astronomical pace. I was awarded Woman of the Year from the National Association of Professional Women; I had speaking engagements and was noted in helped with company training manuals. Women looked up to me and I in turn looked up to them. I think my biggest accomplishment was being asked to speak at a convention in Las Vegas.

I was invited to speak at "The Time is Now Conference" about how I got through my struggles and how I did it all while growing my business. So, thinking about what to talk about I decide to talk about how important it was to have a daily plan in place, planning and setting goals and how that got me through my cancer and kept my business afloat. See, there is a formula on how to get your daily plan done in a short amount of time.

They wanted me to stand before two hundred and fifty people and tell my story. I spoke of how I had a breakthrough and accomplished six figures from my bed. The key is, you have to plug in daily with a specific formula. If I can do this business, anyone can. There are no excuses to building the right business.

After my arrival at the hotel, I joined a few of the conference attendees for a bite to eat. Some of the ladies I knew personally, and some were through social media. It was more than eating a meal together; it was a roundtable of learning and deep discussion.

It was very inspiring! This is just the beginning of an incredible future. Just meeting the ladies in person, all from networking online was an amazing experience within itself. If I never joined Facebook, I would have never been connected to such a dynamic group of women.

Even though standing before that many people was my biggest fear in life, I overcame it. I stood before those people and poured my heart and soul out, on why a daily plan is so important. I teach this to my friends and team. Being prepared for the future and looking at the big picture as you never know what life has in store for you.

Late summer seemed to be a transition time, a growing time. My dad almost lost his life due to neglect in hospitals and nursing homes. My mom and I spent many days by his side; making sure things were done right at these facilities. I also spent four days in the hospital due to flying back from my Las Vegas trip and having blood clots while on the plane.

My ankle and leg blew up just a few hours into the flight. I knew as soon as I got off the plane I needed to head to the hospital. It was confirmed and they needed to admit me as it was not looking good. Thoughts of a surgery to insert a filter into my groin were present but thank God he took care of me and I didn't need it.

I had my computer close by my side during this time. I did hangouts with my team and continued to hit social media pretty hard. I received special messages from my family & friends as they rallied around.

I had my computer close by my side during this time. I did hangouts with my team and continued to hit social media pretty hard.

My business grew so fast. I was award **from National Association of Professional Women** the *Women of the*

Year Award, in company training manuals, had speaking engagements, a wonderful team of people who looked up to me and I looked up to them. I think my biggest accomplishment was being asked to speak at a convention in Las Vegas.

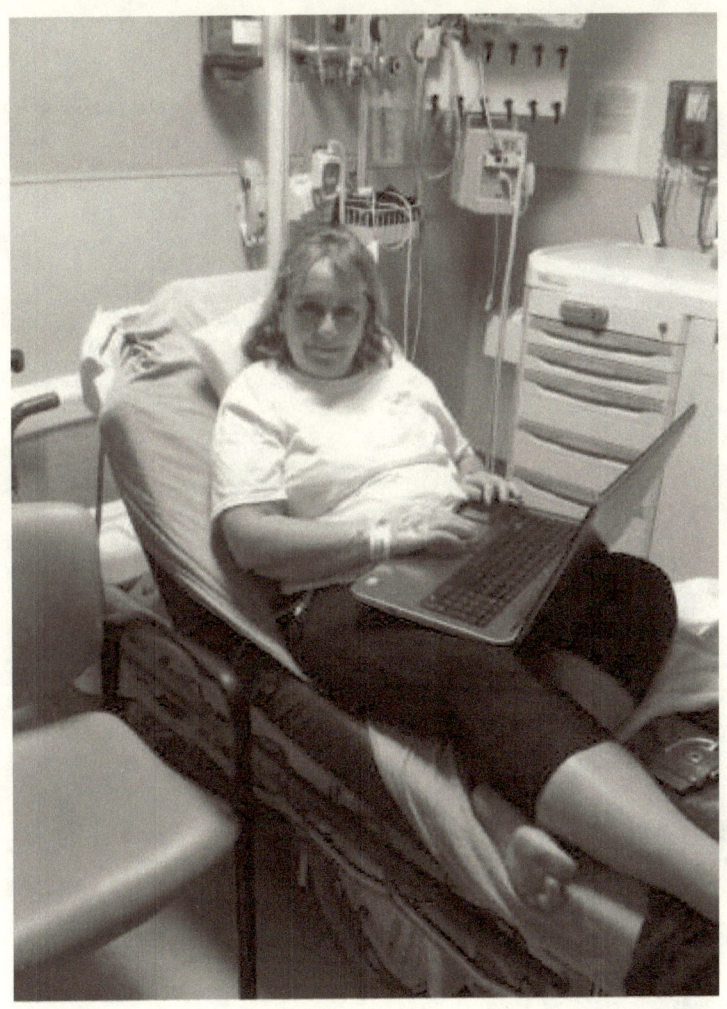

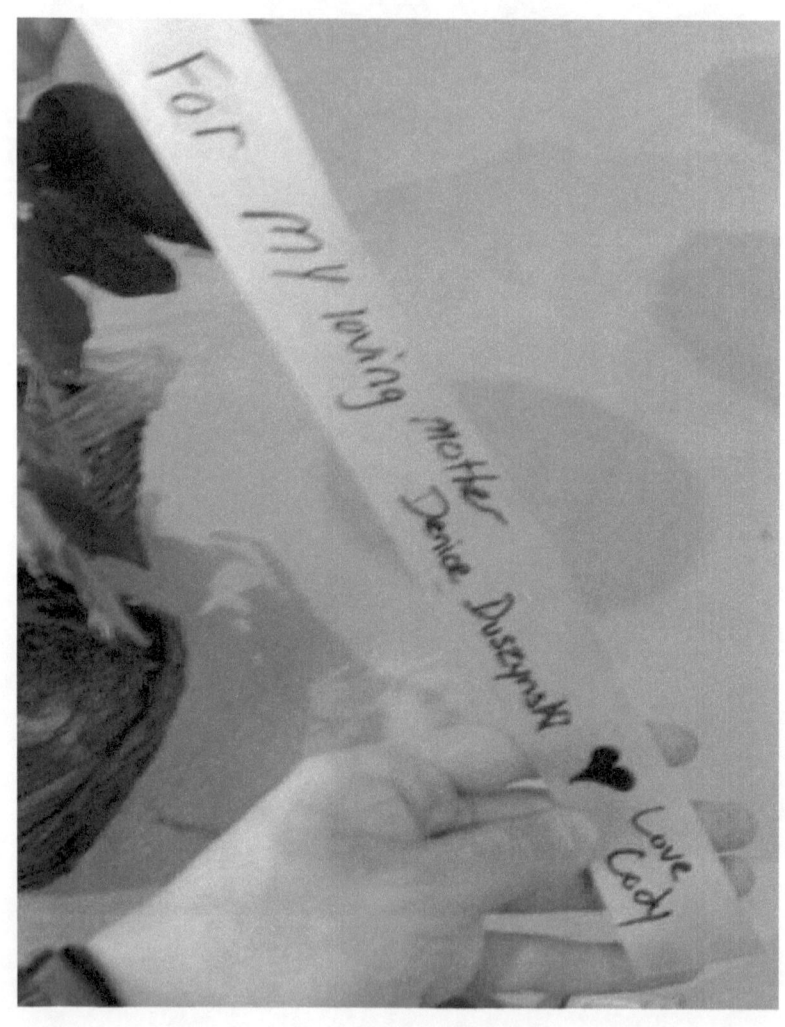

Then something happened on Facebook. No engagement. Social media took a hit. Businesses all over started to decline with everyone that I knew due to the new algorithms. I had been doing the same thing day after day, but the reach was not there. I had to figure out a new way. I have a NO EXCUSE ATTITIDE POLICY. If you say you cannot, you cannot, change your mindset. If I can do it, you can too! So, in the midst of all of this, I began to focus on my heart, my decline had nothing to do with social media, it was me. My heart was not in my business like it was before. The passion had drained from me because of all the betrayals and mismanagement. So, I began to take a look at what was going on.

I explored and searched for answers. I learned of some corporate corruption, the lies and betrayals began. The "big cheeses" were so nice to your face but behind the scenes, they were stacking, moving lines and padding certain people with leads, sales and sales which should have been distributed evenly and equitably during certain promotions.

Corporate emails were being sent to my customers, leading them back to corporate websites, which amounted to losing thousands of sales and clients. Corporate was also developing other businesses and hiding it by putting it in other big network leader's names, hiding it from the public. Why was this happening? Why were so many people not seeing the big picture? Money and greed. It was not about helping people anymore.

I foresaw the demise of the company and the castle began to crumble. This is why I have expanded my businesses. One thing I have learned over the years is to brand yourself and not a product, plus not to put all your eggs in one basket. So, in all the development, a new business was born, Inspired Divas Network... teaching you how to look and feel your best on the inside and out.

During that time, my father became very ill due to medical errors. It started on Christmas Eve 2013, a year ago. He began having chronic looping seizures, seizures that do not stop. I watched with agony, as he left in the ambulance plugged full of IV's and meds on the way to the hospital.

He was the strongest man in my life and the focal point of our family. He was a machinist and a dairy farmer, and he could do or fix anything, even a broken heart. When he was not around life seemed to fall apart.

I watched for months as my dad went in and out of nursing homes and endured the hospital experimenting with the seizure meds taking him to a comatose state. He was not able to function and at one point my father slept thirty days straight. We begged the hospital doctors to reduce the meds levels as he did not show up to the hospital like that. This went on for a year. We fought to bring him home against the hospitals and doctors' recommendations.

They removed all his services because it was against their orders. They thought they were setting us up for failure. I knew we were doing the right thing, and there was a way around this. See, they did not know me. I always know there is a way with God on my side. So, I told my mom as soon as we get him home, we would call his doctor and get him a quick appointment.

I knew once we explained what was going on his doctor would reinstate home health services of a nurses, aids, and physical therapist would be reinstated to come into the house. At that point, dad was very weak. My mom and I struggled to get him in and out of my van; he was dead weight and wheelchair bound. I had to lift him into the vehicle and position him.

We were able to get him to his doctor and back home. It was an exhausting day, but a good day of triumph. All services were reinstated and even our doctor stated what the hospital had done was not right. Again, we felt it was a money game. We are so glad to have my dad home, and he is doing well. He is regaining his strength day by day and very happy to be back in his home.

These are just a few examples of why I have stood firm in my beliefs. I realized I cannot let anyone rob me of my dreams nor can I stand by and let someone do that to someone else's life. If I've learned anything from my journey, it is to be strong, be a voice, and be an advocate for myself and others. Looking back, I realized everything I do is a process, and there's a start, middle, and end. It is like pruning the vine so that new growth can begin. I need to have an attitude of gratitude and believe God has a plan for me. It may not be my plan, but His is the right plan.

I know there's another dimension to my life; I just want to hold my hand out and reach right through to the other side, stepping thru that *Shattered Mirror that Looking Glass.*

I am strong and a survivor and because of this I know I can do anything. The most important thing I can tell you is not to put off today and trade it in for tomorrow. Do it today as you are not promised tomorrow.

Picking up the Pieces after Cancer

Remember that there are people out there that are rooting for you, you just have to find them. If you do not any anyone in your personal life that is supporting you, I urge you to give social media a try. There are people out there that you have not met yet that can be your very best friend. You have access to amazing people, but you have to go out there and find them.

Joy and love to you all today.

PART THREE MY THOUGHTS ON MOTHERHOOD DURING THE CANCER JOURNEY

MOTHERHOOD THROUGH A KALEIDOSCOPE

Motherhood comes in all shapes, sizes and dimensions. It's a Kaleidoscope in 3D! Viewing it is an observation of beautiful forms and distorted colors.

Most of us think of motherhood as having kids and raising them up to be functioning adults in society. It has been a fascinating journey to say the least. I've found that Motherhood is much more than that and comes at so many different levels.

As I reflect over the past four-years, I look back on being a mom and the experiences of having children at a young age.

When you are diagnosed with cancer, you start looking hard at your mortality and who it will affect most; for me, that would be my children.

I know I'm in remission but want to make sure I leave them with a legacy of love and wisdom. I believe love letters and life letters are the best way. So, I continue to journal and write on what to do and when to do it and pray that everything I write will let them know how much I love them.

When I think of motherhood, I think of unconditional love. Motherhood means many things to each individual, and our own definition of it is largely defined by our individual experiences. To one person, motherhood might simply mean the act of raising children; to another, motherhood might be what defines them; for me, it is the deep connection, beyond birthing a child. It's been a kaleidoscope of emotions simultaneously – fear, joy, worry, angst, and so, much pride.

I started out as a young mom, pregnant at 17, which is not an easy road. I was determined to finish high school, and I did.

I returned to school in my senior year, only to hear nasty remarks, feel the weight of unbearable stares, and experience the abandonment of those I thought were friends, who clearly were no longer. I was unable to participate in things that I had planned on in my senior year like cheer, rifle club, and skiing club was out, too. I was fortunate to have a small group of friends around to help me through this; my brother, his friend Randy, who was & is like a brother to me, and a few select friends. They helped me in crowded hallways and made sure I got to class okay.

January to April went by fast and 2-days before my 18th birthday I delivered a healthy 7lb, 7 oz., baby boy. I love this little guy unconditionally. My parents were there for me and helped us through this journey. They were 2nd parents to my 2 youngest children. This was a whole new dimension of life for me. Sharing parenting showed me what unconditional love was.

They loved and cared for my babies like they were their own but still giving us the space to be our own family. I'm forever grateful to my Mom and Dad.

I've been the biggest advocate for my children, empowering them to engage in society in a meaningful, fun, and vibrant way. I've always told them when in search for a career, find one that you will love, that drives your passion and fulfills your purpose. Above all, I have shown them through it all, how to have fun, and that is what they have done.

Four-years ago, I was diagnosed with a rare breast cancer; Triple Negative Aggressive Ductile Cancer, which is not fed on hormones. A five-year survival rate tends to be lower for triple-negative breast cancer as the years go by, but I am beating the odds and with God by my side, I intend to continue living fully, loving my family, and beating cancer.

A 2007 study of more than 50,000 women with all stages of breast cancer found that 77% of women with triple-negative breast cancer survived at least 5-years, versus 93% of women with other types of breast cancer. I have a higher rate of return because of the type of cancer I have, and my solid resolve to live. I have recently had my

Picking up the Pieces after Cancer

BRCA testing updated as they've found new gene studies. More has been revealed.

I have been identified with two cancer genes for colon and ovarian cancers, which are associated with one gene marker, and also lobular breast which is not the kind of cancer I had. Now, this doesn't mean that I have cancer, but with this information I can make more deliberate decisions about my care, and prevention. My family also now has the right to be tested without having insurance companies deny or refuse them access.

So, this is more a love letter to my family than anything else. For me, motherhood didn't just stop at the wonderful children I have. As a result of my own three, James (37), Jessica (35) and Cody (21), I have been blessed with seven grandchildren now, too.

The greatest realization of motherhood for me is that my children are exactly the witty, creative and loving people they are because I was looking for proof that I have done something right. My children are people I love to have around me because they make me laugh, they are cool and interesting, imaginative and fun, and each of them are complete individuals with a unique personality, potential, and talent; and luckily, each has a beautiful, outlook on life. I want my children to always think of fun and family when they think of me.

As a single working mother when my two oldest were young children, I didn't have much time to reflect on much – that stage of my life was pretty much dedicated to surviving; paying bills and putting food on the table. I missed my kids so much when they were little. It was always my dream to work from home and be with them. No matter what I did, it never happened back then. Computers were just coming into play and social media wasn't even heard of at that time. However, I did find the perfect combination and finally made my breakthrough in working from home and creating a 6-figure income. It was the best. I could schedule everything around my family and be home. Now when my kids call for help or want to spend time with me or I want some extra time with the grandkids, I can drop everything and do what I love most; be the best mom and grandma ever!

Jamie has two girls ages 10 and 14 and it is so much fun when they are around. I take pride that they always help me with household tasks when I'm not up to it. I'm so proud of Jamie as he's a hard worker and a great provider for his family; a bit of a work-a-holic, with passion for his hobbies.

In the spring he makes maple syrup, and in the summer, he has a huge garden. He's always researching and creating gizmos and gadgets. He recently made a home version of a sawmill and also took up carving wood. He did a beautiful version of a hummingbird in a morning glory; always something creative on his mind. He's also taken on the responsibility of his wife's two kids. He's such an awesome Dad and has grown into a fine young man. I do think that my medical issues scared my oldest, as he didn't come around much during my treatments.

I know I am in his heart but because he is such a sensitive soul, he couldn't bear to see what I was going through. I watched you grow and grow, over the years. I still remember when you were little; you hated to wear your pants and would run around without them on. You were full of life and so much fun. I've always called you 'my little genius'!

My daughter Jessica was a leg hugger as a toddler. When she was little, she would hide behind me and hug my legs when people were around. She hated strangers and would cling to me like glue. She was an adventurous tike though, playing in oil and graphite getting it all over her new clothes, 'to make pretty colors'! Today she is an artist and has a deep passion for people. Her artwork is the most imaginative things I've ever seen. She works in mixed media and does 3-D paintings. Jessica is also an LPN and has worked with disabled adults and seniors. During my chemo, she came out weekly to give me my shots to build my bone marrow and help me heal. She too, is a life-giver.

Picking up the Pieces after Cancer

I thank God for her every day, because traveling to get this done would have been too much for me. Her heart and soul are generous and kind, and she would do anything for you. During my cancer journey, she was supportive and also put on a "Strike Out Cancer" benefit for me. I'm grateful and so appreciative for this, as it helped me keep my insurance and pay my bills. Jess is also a stepmom to a young boy. I'm happy that she is such a good mom. Her quick and amusing responses will have you rolling on the floor laughing.

My youngest son, Cody was my handful. At a young age he was diagnosed with Oppositional Defiance Disorder (ODD), Attention deficit and Hyperactivity Disorder (ADHD), Intermittent Explosive Disorder (IED), and Severe Depression. That in itself was a taxing for everyone, but a journey that brought us closer together. Sometimes I felt that I was the only one that understood his pain. When people look at you on the outside and don't know what's going on in the inside, the just think there's something wrong with you. There was a lot of judgment.

He has a legitimate neurological disorder and his brain waves go haywire sometimes.

He appeared out-of-control, but with patience, compassion, love, and groundbreaking research and collaboration with experts, I'm proud to say that my Cody is a normal young man that has taken on the world to be the best person he can be.

Cody has met a wonderful young woman with two little girls of her own. Those babies, I love more than anything. They have brought me much love and joy over the past year that I could ever imagine. When I arrive at their house, **Miss Molli** can't wait to come down the stairs and cries anxiously waiting for me to pick her up. She is just 2 years old. I've never had a connection with someone like this before. She's my little love. I cherish every moment we have together. Her sister is 2-years older and she's such a little doll. She has a smile that would light up you heart at any given moment.

Picking up the Pieces after Cancer

There is great vulnerability in knowing that I have today only. That every choice I have made from before my children were born right up to this moment, is the sum total of a life that will someday come to an end. I know I have impacted my children. I've done some good stuff. I'm proud to say, "It's always the mother's fault." I just know that as the time passes, I get more credit than blame for how my children turned out. I am so proud to be emotionally invested in the results, and equally exhausted by the labor of it all; strangely confident that it will all, turn out okay.

Motherhood is job for which there is no practice. There is no duplicatable training, you just sort of learn on the job and take each 'project' as it comes. Like all moms, I know that I've made mistakes, and pushed too, hard many times, and sometimes I know I did not push nearly hard enough. But I can honestly say that I have done my job and I have done it with all I had to give.

I imagine you've all felt neglected or unimportant at times when my attention seemed focused elsewhere, and at times one of you needed my attention more than the other, but I have always been there, watching, and sometimes letting you have the room to struggle and do for yourselves. Mothers do that, too, you know. It is hardest to stand back, but when success came, they were yours to own. I thank God for giving me little respites here and there, and for helping me survive all the childhood hurts. I've stretched my heart in ways I never knew were possible.

It's how you love through the ups and downs, the challenges that life brings. And, it lasts a lifetime from that first tiny cry.

As the quote from Elizabeth Stone goes, *"having a child is to decide forever to have your heart go walking around outside your body."*

Picking up the Pieces after Cancer

Each of my children and grandchildren has turned out to be the most delightful people you will ever meet in your life and I know my heart will be walking this planet, long after I am gone.

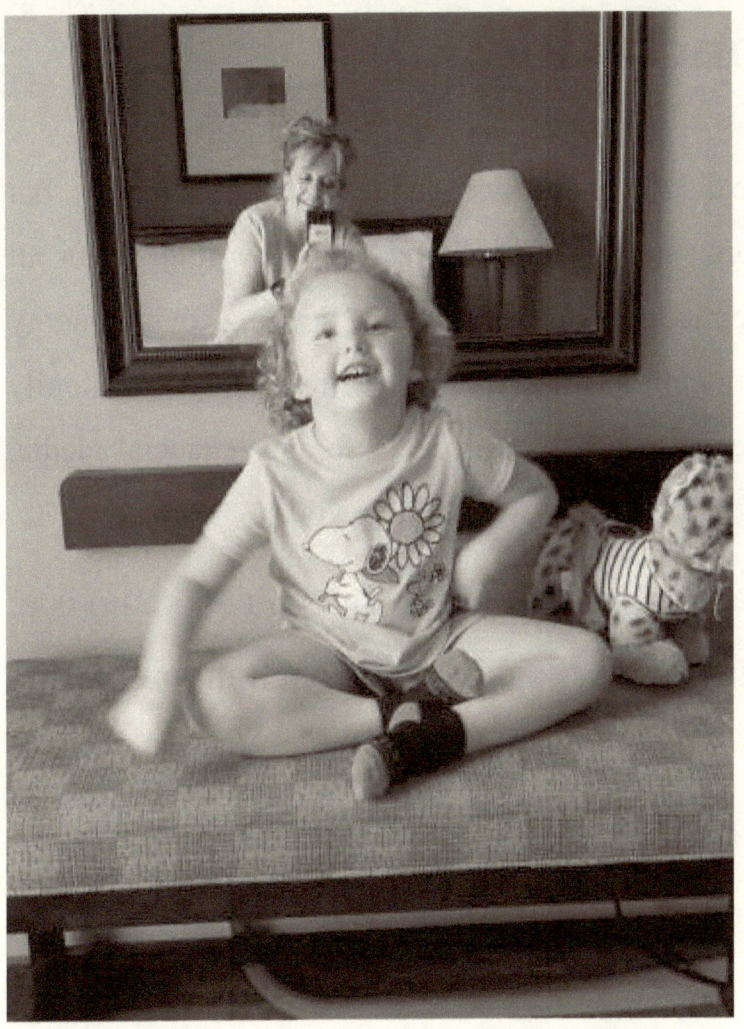

Little Miss Mollie – My Little Angel

Conclusion:

The diagnosis of cancer can take your breath away, but it can only steal as much life as you allow it to. Focus all of your thoughts on being healed sending loving energy into your cells as they repair and rejuvenate. Allow family and friends to help you in real life and on social media. Virtual friends really want to help you.

Remember that every day you wake up is a new day to start again. Take each moment as it comes to you.

Contact Information

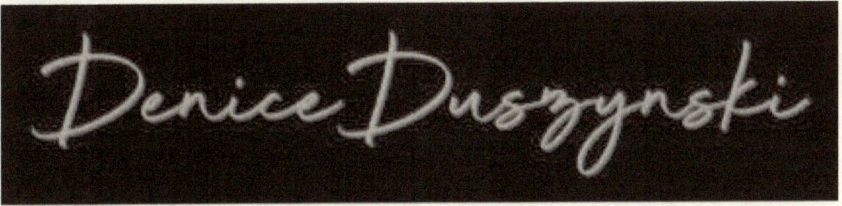

Email: coachdenice@gmail.com

Facebook: @ DeniceMDuszynski

Website: InspiredSocialDiva.com

Picking up the Pieces after Cancer